HealthyDimensions™
Program Workbook

Elizabeth Wright RN, MSN

Dedication

This workbook is dedicated to all the men and women
who have spent years, or even lifetimes
struggling with their weight.

People who've gotten bad advice
and inadequate support for
both the body and the mind.

May the Healthy Dimensions process
and your personal journey
bring you to a place of
health and inner peace.

Limitations of the Healthy Dimensions™ program

The Healthy Dimensions program materials and website provide education about options to help participants lose weight and improve their overall health. You are responsible for your own choices about which options to adopt. You must consider your choices carefully and should obtain advice from trusted healthcare providers about any concerns that you have.

Participants who are taking medications MUST be managed by a physician. Rapid weight loss and relief of water retention may drastically reduce the appropriate dose for anti-diabetic and anti-hypertensive drugs. Blood pressure or blood sugar could become dangerously low. The effectiveness and safety of other medications may also change with weight loss. You take full responsibility for discussing this program and weight loss goals with your physician and arranging for adequate follow up with your physician for potential changes in medication doses.

Persons with kidney disease may not be allowed to follow the standard dietary recommendations in this program. If you have been diagnosed with kidney disease, you agree to not make any dietary changes that are unless they are supported by your physician.

Healthy Dimensions is not intended to provide medical advice. All information, content, and materials are for informational purposes only and are not intended to serve as a substitute for the consultation, diagnosis, and/or medical treatment of a qualified physician or healthcare provider.

IF YOU BELIEVE YOU HAVE A MEDICAL EMERGENCY, YOU SHOULD IMMEDIATELY CALL 911 OR YOUR PHYSICIAN. If you believe you have any other health problem, or if you have any questions regarding your health or a medical condition, you should promptly consult your physician or other healthcare provider. Never disregard medical or professional advice, or delay seeking it, because of something you have learned in the Healthy Dimensions program or read on the website

Table of Contents

How to use this workbook _____ 9

Week 1 – Why We're Here (HD Chapter 1) _____ 11
   Creating motivation _____ 11
   Chapter content _____ 13
   Assignment for the week _____ 14

Week 2 – Transforming Metabolism (HD Chapter 2) _____ 15
   Report out _____ 15
   Chapter content _____ 16
   Evaluate for insulin resistance _____ 17
   The Metabolic Healing Diet_____ 19
      TRACK Personal Nutrition and Lifestyle Plan_____ 20
   Fabulous foods to eat on my plan _____ 24
      Breakfast _____ 24
      Lunch _____ 25
      Dinner _____ 26
      Snacks _____ 27
   Support for common symptoms _____ 29
      TRACK symptoms _____ 30
   Favorite low-carb dishes_____ 31
      Breakfast _____ 31
      Lunch or dinner_____ 33
      Snacks _____ 37
   Assignment for the week _____ 39
   Growth Opportunities_____ 39

Week 3 – Willpower (HD Chapter 3) _____ 41
   Report out_____ 41
   Chapter content _____ 42
   Willpower and the depletion of mental energy _____ 43
   Willpower tools _____ 45
      Avoid temptation _____ 46
      Exercise willpower muscles _____ 47
      Silence the inner nag _____ 48
      Make powerful goals _____ 49
      A line in the sand: Boundaries _____ 50
      Make a plan: Clear and flexible _____ 51
      Share and compare _____ 51
      Self-awareness_____ 52
   Changing the food monolog _____ 53
   Make a plan for changing the chatter in your mind about food _____ 54
      Control stress chemicals _____ 54

Notice the negative bias of your brain _____ 55
This is not me, this is my creation _____ 55
Simulate success with food challenges _____ **57**
TRACK simulating for success _____ 59
Assignment for the week _____ **60**
Growth Opportunities _____ **60**

Week 4 – Food Sensitivities and Hunger-vs-Desire (HD Chapters 4 & 5) _____ **63**
Report out _____ **63**
Chapter content _____ **64**
Considering food sensitivities in your Personal Nutrition and Lifestyle Plan ____ **64**
TRACK food sensitivity trails _____ 66
Wheat and addictive exorphins _____ **67**
Hunger vs. desire? _____ **69**
Feed the need: Awesome alternatives to food _____ **71**
TRACK I Wanna Eat log _____ 73
End emotional eating: Changing your mind and choosing beliefs _____ **75**
Programs and beliefs for future analysis _____ **77**
Assignment for the week _____ **78**
Growth Opportunities _____ **78**

Week 5 – Stress and Choosing Beliefs (HD Chapter 6) _____ **81**
Report out _____ **81**
Chapter content _____ **82**
Identifying the stress response _____ **83**
TRACK the stress response _____ 84
Identifying stressors _____ **85**
Should-ing on yourself and powerful choices _____ **87**
Changing your mind about stressors _____ **89**
Work through tough stressors – Dig into beliefs _____ **91**
TRACK progress on stress _____ 95
Love yourself _____ **96**
TRACK how often you are good to yourself _____ 97
Assignment for the week _____ **98**
Growth Opportunities _____ **98**

Week 6 – Inflammation and Happiness (HD Chapters 7 & 8) _____ **101**
Report out _____ **101**
Do I have chronic inflammation? _____ **103**
Reversing inflammation _____ **105**
Alcohol _____ **105**
TRACK response to alcohol _____ 106
Happiness _____ **107**
Gratitude _____ 107
Optimism _____ 109
Create flow experiences _____ 110
Assignment for the week _____ **111**

Growth Opportunities_____ 111
Week 7 – Maintaining a Healthy Relationship with Food (HD Chapter 9)_____ 115
Report out_____ 115
Chapter content _____ 116
Planning for favorite foods _____ 117
TAME a binge _____ 118
Return to fat metabolism _____ 119
Use the power of an observer _____ 119
Planning for the rest of the journey_____ 121
    Set realistic goals _____ 121
    Fine-tune your nutrition plan _____ 121
    Continue to develop your PNLP _____ 122
Creating an ongoing support group _____ 123

How to use this workbook

How long will this program take?

This self-paced workbook is designed to mimic the original Healthy Dimensions™ Quick Start Workshop, which is completed over 7 weekly two-hour sessions. However, the reader who is using this workbook to follow the Healthy Dimensions program independently, or with their own group, is encouraged to proceed at whatever pace works best. Don't feel limited or pressured by the session labels of "Week 1, 2" etc.

How do I get support?

There's a lot to be gained by talking with fellow travelers about the many concepts and tools you'll be exploring in this workbook. Speaking your plans and challenges to others is a powerful evidence-based tool for increasing success in major life changes.

Why not develop or join a virtual or in-person group and discover your healthy dimensions together? Even having just one person to bounce things off will increase your commitment, and evidence shows it will also increase your chances of success.

If you're teaming up with a group or a buddy, each of the exercises is an opportunity for discussion, along with self-reflection. Go through them in order and take the time to allow each member to contribute to the conversation.

You may find each "weekly" session here works better as two sessions for you or your group. Or you may power through the material at lightning speed. See what the group/buddy wants and be flexible.

Many options for getting support are available at the Healthy-Dimensions.com website. From simply joining the online networking groups to getting personalized 1:1 coaching, whatever level of support you need is available.

You may uncover some deeply buried thoughts or beliefs in this process and working with a trusted counselor or even a professional therapist might help keep you moving forward toward your weight loss goals. You are encouraged to get help and support if you seem to be getting stuck anywhere.

What is the structure?

The exercises in this workbook are created with the assumption that you've read the associated chapter(s) in the Healthy Dimensions book. Many important concepts are introduced there.

Remember that this program introduces a starting place for a way of eating and that an important part of the Healthy Dimensions process is developing your own unique mind/body plan. The "perfect approach" for weight loss is a very individual thing.

The Healthy Dimensions program provides many evidence-based mind/body tools designed to help you succeed and a structure to start applying them in your life. Explore these tools with an open mind, and then pick and choose only those that feel right and work for YOU. These tools are then added to your Personal Nutrition and Lifestyle Plan (PNLP).

Tracking your progress and the details of your PNLP are a critical ingredient to winning at losing weight. Research has shown that tracking increases the likelihood of success.

As you move through the process with this workbook and the Healthy Dimensions book, examples of tracking tools are offered; no particular method is required. Tailor your method of tracking to your lifestyle, but it is essential that you do it in some way.

The more you engage in this discovery process, the more likely you'll succeed.

Carefully considering the questions and trying out the tools in this workbook will give you a framework for discovering your perfect combination of mind/body changes so that weight loss becomes perfectly natural. Along the way you will have the opportunity to discover an increased sense of power and control in your experience of life.

This process is worth your time.
You are worth this time.
How much time are you willing to give yourself every day to find your healthy dimensions?

Good luck on your transformative journey!

Week 1 – Why We're Here (HD Chapter 1)

The most important part of making any life change is motivation. This is one thing that can't be provided by any weight loss program; it has to come from within. Before you begin this process, set the stage and get excited!

Although this may be the most comfortable weight loss program you've ever known, it will still take some attention and sometimes it will be challenging. Really wanting the prize at the end, deeply desiring whatever you get when you are at a healthy weight, is essential. Take some time to thoughtfully consider the following:

Creating motivation

My goals are:

1.

2.

3.

Reaching these goals benefits me in these ways:

Short term

Long term

Reaching these goals benefits other people in my life in these ways:

Short term

Long term

Pick an event in the next 12 months and write in detail about how amazing it will be to be thinner and healthier at this event. Really put yourself there and feel the experience.

Event:

Date:

What it will be like physically and emotionally:

List 3 ways to make this goal bigger and more present in your day-to-day life.
(e.g., write about it, talk about it, post it on your wall, Photoshop your face onto a thinner body and print it off, etc.)

1.

2.

3.

Which of these ways are you willing to commit to doing?

Chapter content

What resonated with you?

What surprised you?

What is your emotional response to this information and why?

How does this information change any self-recrimination or guilt you may be carrying related to why you're overweight?

Assignment for the week

1. Do NOT change your diet until you have read Chapter 2 in the book and completed week 2 in the workbook.
2. Choose a method to start tracking what you eat. You will want to know, at minimum, your daily intake of calories as well as grams and % of fat, carbohydrate, and protein. Start tracking before you change your diet, at least for a few days, so you get practice and more importantly, know your current intake for later comparison.
3. Track down recent lab work, including lipid and metabolic panels that show fasting blood glucose, HDL/LDL cholesterol, and triglycerides.
   - ✓ If you haven't had this routine blood work done in the last year, please schedule an appointment to have it done.
   - ✓ It is important to know your starting place. These labs are also discussed in the next session.

Week 2 – Transforming Metabolism (HD Chapter 2)

Report out

What was it like to track your intake?

What did you learn about your current eating patterns?

What are your current lab values for the following?

_____HDL cholesterol

_____LDL cholesterol

_____VLDL cholesterol (if available)

_____Triglycerides

_____Fasting blood glucose

What are your thoughts about these lab values?

Chapter content

What did you learn about the physiology of metabolism that you didn't already know?

What resonated with you?

What surprised you?

Do you think your body has been in the carb-hunger cycle?

What if your weight problems have been caused by excess insulin rather than from personal weakness? How does this change things for you?

Evaluate for insulin resistance

Now that you understand more about your metabolism and the dangers of excess insulin, do you think you're at risk for the health effects of excess insulin and ultimately insulin resistance?

How many family members had the following diseases associated with insulin resistance/metabolic syndrome?

___Obesity
___Diabetes
___Heart disease (heart attack, congestive heart failure)
___Vascular disease (including arteriosclerosis and hypertension)
___Stroke
___Fatty liver disease
___Cancers of the breast, colon, gall bladder, kidney, and possibly prostate
___Psoriasis
___Polycystic ovary syndrome
___Premature "cognitive" aging (dementia / Alzheimer's)

A combination of any THREE of the following symptoms is needed for a medical diagnosis of metabolic syndrome.

Which do you have?

☐ Increased abdominal fat - experts offer different ways to define it:

- Some use actual waist size, 40" for men and 35" for women (smaller measurements for people of Asian descent).
- Some use a waist-to-hip ratio – that is, waist measurement divided by hip measurement. A measurement above .9 for men and above .85 for women indicates abdominal obesity.
- The World Health Organization (WHO) says any BMI level of over 30.

☐ An elevated fasting insulin level

☐ Triglycerides over 150 milligrams per deciliter (mg/dL)

☐ HDL – anything below 40 mg/dL in men and below 50 mg/dL in women

☐ Elevated blood pressure – anything greater than 130/85

☐ Fasting blood glucose over 100 mg/dL

Are you at risk for the diseases of insulin resistance?

How does this assessment affect the list of benefits you started last week?

Turn back to the Motivation section and add the potential health benefits if you

- ✓ reduce your insulin
- ✓ start burning your own fat
- ✓ stop living in the carb-hunger cycle

These benefits may be an important aspect of developing strong motivation!

The Metabolic Healing Diet

What are your thoughts about trying this approach to eating?

An overview of the recommended dietary approach follows. This very low-carb way of eating is likely to minimize insulin in even the most resistant metabolisms. Note that over time you may choose to increase your total NET carbs until your weight loss stops or cravings return.

1. No sugar, grains, soy, or alcohol for the first 4 weeks. Many people have bodies that are sensitive to these items; you will add them back later and evaluate your response to them.
2. Any other foods or beverages are acceptable within the following guideline:
   - Consume </=20 grams of NET carbohydrate daily.
   - NET = total carb grams minus fiber grams.
3. Daily minimum of 2 cups green vegetables is strongly recommended.
4. Calculate and consume at least your minimum daily protein requirement (there are many online options for calculating this requirement).
5. Track your weight and calories, fat, protein, and NET carb grams. It is helpful to know the percentage of fat, protein and carbs as well. My Fitness Pal and Fit Day meet these expectations, and many others are available.
   - Aim for at least 60% fat and adjust for feelings of satisfaction and weight loss.
   - Don't worry about calories at this time but eat when hungry and stop when satisfied.

After 2 weeks,

1. Begin to increase carbohydrate intake gradually if desired (some prefer to stay at 20 grams of carbs until they reach their goal weight).
   - Increase carbohydrates to 25 grams/day in the third week, 30 grams/day in fourth week, etc. until weight loss stops or cravings return.

- Decrease to the number of grams/day that produced weight loss and eliminated cravings.
2. Continue to develop and follow your Personal Nutrition & Lifestyle Plan (PNLP) until you have reached goal weight.
3. To get past plateaus, try one of these options for several days at a time – and return to tracking if you have stopped!
    - Increase fat % or decrease protein % in diet.
    - Reduce carbohydrates (it is OK to go below 20 grams/day if that helps keep hunger at bay).
    - Some people lose better with more calories, some with less, so experiment with total calories to determine your optimal weight loss combination.

Adding variety (wait at least 4 weeks)
1. Add alcohol sparingly. Complete session 6 in this workbook before adding it back into your lifestyle. Some people cannot lose weight when consuming alcohol, some can.
2. Re-introduce sugar, grains, and soy individually and incrementally, watching carefully for weight and physical responses. Complete session 4 in this workbook before reintroducing them.

Maintenance at goal weight

As weight drops, you'll discover what your body needs to be at a normal weight. It's not going to change much from how you were eating the day you reached your goal. You will not go back to eating the way you do now. Which, by then, won't be such a big deal because you will find this way of eating is delicious and satisfying.

If your weight increases by 5 pounds, return to recording all dietary intake and follow your PNLP closely until weight normalizes. If you are aware and tracking, you'll learn your limits and find the balance.

TRACK Personal Nutrition and Lifestyle Plan

The next page is an example tracking form you might use as you develop your Personal Nutrition and Lifestyle Plan (PNLP) over the next several weeks; it includes the key items to track. You might copy this and fill it out by hand, make something similar as an Excel file, or use any other tracking option.

Personal Nutrition & Lifestyle Plan (PNLP) Tracking Sheet

Dietary Goals	Lifestyle Goals	Date	Cal	Intake Carb gm	Carb %	Fat %	Pro %	Significant Activities / Comments	Sense of well-being 0-10	Level of craving 1-10	Weight next morning

Personal Nutrition & Lifestyle Plan (PNLP) Tracking Sheet

Dietary Goals	Lifestyle Goals		Intake						Significant Activities / Comments	Sense of well-being 0-10	Level of craving 1-10	Weight next morning
		Date	Cal	Carb gm	Carb %	Fat %	Pro %					

Personal Nutrition & Lifestyle Plan (PNLP) Tracking Sheet

Dietary Goals	Lifestyle Goals	Date	Intake						Significant Activities / Comments	Sense of well-being 0-10	Level of craving 1-10	Weight next morning
			Cal	Carb g()	Carb %	Fat %	Pro %					

Fabulous foods to eat on my plan

Some ideas for delicious meals are included below under "Favorite low carb dishes." Read through these and/or go online and start exploring low-carb recipes, or buy a low-carb cookbook. Fill out the following list with as many ideas as you can. When you're wondering what to eat, come back to this list.

Breakfast

1.

2.

3.

4.

5.

6.

7.

8.

9.

10.

11.

12.

Lunch

1.

2.

3.

4.

5.

6.

7.

8.

9.

10.

11.

12.

13.

14.

15.

16.

Dinner

1.

2.

3.

4.

5.

6.

7.

8.

9.

10.
.

11.

12.

13.

14.

15.

16.

Snacks

1.

2.

3.

4.

5.

6.

7.

8.

9.

10.
.
11.

12.

13.

14.

15.

16.

Other delicious foods I will enjoy:

Support for common symptoms

During the shift from carbohydrate to fat-burning metabolism, you may experience some side effects for a few days. Carefully review this section in the book again.

Dehydration, low sodium, and low potassium – treatment is CRITICAL!!

These symptoms are caused by the excretion of water as insulin levels decrease. The electrolytes that are excreted MUST be replaced.

Symptoms:
- Leg cramps
- Headaches
- Dizziness
- Nausea
- Fatigue
- Irritability
- Palpitations

Treatment:
- ✓ Drink plenty of water. Remember, caffeine increases water loss.
- ✓ Eat salty foods, use salt liberally, and/or drink bouillon 1-2 x day.
- ✓ Eat potassium-rich foods, and use supplements as needed.

Note here what symptoms you experience during the shift to fat metabolism, how you treat them, and your body's response (tracker provided on the next page).

TRACK symptoms

Date/time	Symptom	Treatment/response

Favorite low-carb dishes

A bird's eye view of the many delicious foods that are available with a low-carb way of eating.

Many people find that cooking some favorites ahead of time makes it easy to have something to "grab and go" throughout the week.

Breakfast

Great any time of the day!

Scramble

Mix eggs with heavy cream, melt butter in pan, sauté at low heat until about ¾ cooked, add one or more of the following, stir occasionally until eggs are almost done, top with cheese and cover until nicely melted. Serve with sour cream... and hot sauce!

All of these ingredients are better when sautéed to golden before adding to the eggs, if you have the time. You can cook up a bunch and keep them in the fridge ready to throw on the eggs any morning.
- Ham
- Sausage
- Bacon
- Pepperoni
- Chopped onions
- Mushrooms
- Zucchini
- Green beans - any leftover low-carb vegetable

Eggs Benedict

Just skip the muffin and have some extra Canadian bacon! I like the Betty Crocker recipe for Hollandaise, just butter, lemon, and an egg. Follow the recipe and don't walk away...keep stirring!

Meat roll-ups

Fairly thick sliced roast beef or ham or turkey spread with cream cheese and garlic salt, Italian spices, and shredded parmesan - roll 'em up alone or with a big lettuce leaf.

Alternately, roll with American, provolone, or any other cheese and add what sounds good – like jalapenos or sautéed mushrooms or hot sauce or mayo instead of the cream cheese. Good for breakfast or anytime.

Lettuce-wich

Big lettuce leaves really are a great thing to hold a hamburger (it's a bit drippy but who cares?) or with any sandwich fillers. It gives you that hand-to-mouth feeling, which is just nice and normal. How about a BLT? Use plenty of bacon – I often keep it in the fridge already cooked. Just put it in the microwave for a few seconds and add some tomato and mayo on a big lettuce leaf (surprisingly gratifying).

Egg salad (with or without meat)

Make up a bunch and it's ready for several days. It's easy to just eat a few spoonfuls out of the fridge for a healthy snack. Very satisfying and simple; eggs are a good base for a variety of options.

Just add mayo and/or mustard to chopped boiled eggs. Consider adding green olives and shrimp, tuna or chicken, onions, celery, or zucchini. Cheddar cheese is a particularly good addition.

Crust-less quiche

In a basic quiche recipe, the liquid base consists of a ratio of 6 eggs per cup of heavy cream; add meats and low-carb vegetables of any kind (make in pie plate or muffin tins). Make these ahead and freeze them; you can microwave them for a few seconds for a quick meal or snack.

Leftovers from dinner

They're quick and easy, nobody says you can't have dinner for breakfast!

Lunch or dinner

Salad as a meal

Salad greens have very few carbs after the fiber is subtracted. Add eggs, cheese, bacon, avocado, onions, chicken, steak, shrimp, nuts – the possibilities are endless. Carefully choose a low-carb dressing or simply mix olive oil and vinegar together for a completely carb-free option. Remember, you don't have to skimp on the dressing anymore!

Veggies

Veggies that are low-carb and yummy: mushrooms, cauliflower, broccoli, spaghetti squash, zucchini or yellow summer squash, onions, eggplant, peppers. Eat them fresh or sauté them with fresh garlic and plenty of butter or olive oil.

Fruits

Many fruits are very high in carbs. Here are some lower-carb suggestions.

- Avocado is a high-fat lower-carb fruit, and it goes with everything.
- Choose berries; raspberries, blueberries, and strawberries pack the biggest punch nutritionally with the fewest carbs. Homemade whipped cream (use calorie-free sweetener) on berries is really satisfying.
- Tomatoes can really make a dish, but they are a fruit and have more carbs than many vegetables. Count the carbs!

Meat

Obviously whole natural meat is carb-free. Remember that protein stimulates insulin to some degree, but also glucagon. It's a shift in thinking but higher fat meats are actually better for a low-carb way of eating. Some high-fat meat options to enjoy include:

- Prime rib when you go out or a rib roast from the grocery store makes any meal special. It has an excellent omega 6/3 profile and you can use the leftovers to make a great quick snack. Cook one for dinner and use for snacks and meals the rest of the week.
- Pot roast is delicious; just substitute whole mushrooms and chunks of colored peppers for the potato and carrots.

- Fresh sausage may seem sinful, but it really isn't. Higher fat meats are actually better for weight loss in the low-carb world, so enjoy! How about Italian sausage and peppers or brats on the grill?
- Ribs are delicious, but be sure to see the BBQ sauce item in the next section.
- Deli meats can contain carbs, so read labels. There is much conflicting evidence about whether processed meats are "bad" for you. Do your own research and make a choice. They do add variety to a low-carb way of eating.
- Seafood really seems like a special treat, especially with butter to dip it in or a nice sauce to ladle on top (see aioli in the next section).
- Cheese dog - cut a hot dog lengthwise and stick a slice of American cheese in the opening. Microwave or broil and cut into 1 inch pieces. Throw on some chopped onion and jalapenos... quick and yummy!
- Cheeseburgers are delicious, and if you add bacon, avocado, onion or other toppings they're even better. Eat with a fork and knife or wrap it up in a lettuce leaf.

Sauces

Many wonderful sauces are low in carbs and make the ingredients above taste a LOT better.

- White sauce. Start with butter and cream and go from there (lemon, dill, garlic, southwestern, oriental, or whatever). To keep carbs low, reduce your sauces with heat and time instead of adding flour or cornstarch. Another option is to thicken with cauliflower sauce.
- Cauliflower sauce. Cook cauliflower in broth until fairly mushy, strain off the broth and whip the cauliflower in a blender – it makes a GREAT thickening agent for a white sauce or cream soup.
- Hollandaise and Béarnaise sauce make everything better.
- BBQ sauce. Many BBQ sauces contain sugar. Some hot sauces are completely carb-free but check labels. Make homemade BBQ sauce starting with low-sugar ketchup (Heinz has one) as a base. There are increasing numbers of sugar-free BBQ sauces in stores.
- Sour cream just makes everything better and is low in carbs (don't buy low-fat sour cream, it has more carbs).
- Aioli is basically any flavored mayonnaise, my favorite is simple: garlic and hot mustard. Anything you can imagine can become an aioli; Cajun, Spanish, Mediterranean, Moroccan – keep one or more in the fridge. Just about any meat can be dipped in aioli, which makes

it different than 'just meat again.' It provides the fat your body needs and makes you feel satisfied.

- Guacamole – well of course! See Chip/cracker substitutes in the "Snacks" section below.

Creamy cheesy casseroles and side dishes

Creamy and cheesy and soft in your mouth, a casserole can really be comfort food. Some vegetables substitute very well for pasta, potatoes, or rice. The cream, cheese, and meat in a casserole are already very low-carb. Mix your desired ingredients together, and bake in a casserole dish until brown and bubbly. Add more cream if it looks too dry. This can also be a quick snack later.

- "Riced" cauliflower. There are recipes online, but basically you can just pulse fresh cauliflower in a food processor to small rice sized pieces, cook covered in the microwave for a couple of minutes, and drain. The consistency to look for is midway between soft and raw. Use as a substitute for rice.
- Cauliflower casserole. Try simply adding chunks of cauliflower as a substitution for potato or pasta in any recipe. Steam or roast to *al dente* before adding to the casserole. A simple cauliflower casserole might include sautéed mushrooms, onions, and garlic. Top with cheese, cream, salt, pepper, and a little nutmeg, then bake until bubbly. Add chicken, ham, or any other meat to make it a meal instead of a side dish. Individual-sized casserole dishes make this feel like a real treat; they are a good investment.
- Broccoli casserole. Broccoli is a natural fit for casseroles. How about broccoli with bits of ham and lots of cheese and cream… add mushrooms here too. Like broccoli rice casserole? See riced cauliflower above.
- "Macaroni" and cheese. Cut zucchini into macaroni-sized pieces and sauté to *al dente* in garlic and butter. Make a cheese sauce from American cheese and cream and pour it over the zucchini. This satisfies the mac and cheese need and soon you'll realize it actually tastes better!

Cauliflower mashed potatoes
Cut cauliflower into chunks, steam until done and drain very well. Mash with butter, cream cheese, and cream. Some like to add nutmeg. This dish is very delicious. Before long you will wonder why you ever wanted potatoes!

Burrito in a bowl

Add seasoned browned hamburger (don't use the seasoning packets, they're loaded with carbs) and chopped tomatoes previously cooked with Mexican spices. Add chopped peppers, onions, and top with cheese. Bake until bubbly. See also guacamole and sour cream in the "Sauces" section above!

Tacos

Wrap your taco ingredients in a lettuce leaf, you really won't miss the shell. Alternately, you could make a taco shell made of fried cheese, which is crispy and delicious. See "frico chips" in the following "Snacks" section.

Pizza as a casserole

Mix homemade/sugar-free marinara with mushrooms, pepperoni, sausage, peppers, and olives. Put it in a shallow single serving baking dish with whole-milk mozzarella on top (it's way better than part-skim). Bake until golden.

Pizza with a cauliflower crust

It sounds weird but it is truly delicious. This crust has the texture and feel of bread and does not taste like cauliflower. Google the recipe. A couple of tips:

- DON'T use whole-milk mozzarella for the crust here, part-skim works better.
- Using half parmesan and half mozzarella is my favorite combination.
- Don't be afraid to add spices and sautéed garlic to the crust "batter."
- Precook the crust until golden, then let it cool.
- Add a little sauce and everything else you want. Putting pepperoni at the bottom will help protect the crust from the moisture of the sauce.
- Top with whole-milk mozzarella and broil until cheese is bubbly, it doesn't take long.

Veal, chicken, or eggplant Parmesan

Pour (sugar-free or homemade) marinara on top of cooked meat and add a slice of whole-milk mozzarella. Bake until golden and bubbly.

- Eggplant is best if dehydrated in a slow oven ahead of time.

- Some pieces of broccoli or red pepper slices could be added to the baking dish for color and flavor.
- You can also "bread" your item with almond meal or almond flour if you like and sauté before putting in the oven.

Pasta sauces

Watch out for spaghetti/marinara sauce from a jar, it's loaded with sugar. The best bet is diced or canned tomatoes cooked down with spices. Consider adding a little artificial sweetener and olive oil. Make a bunch and freeze in Ziploc bags.

Most Alfredo sauces are low in carbohydrates.

Spaghetti or noodles

There are several options to choose from. New lower carb noodle substitutes are showing up in the marketplace; read labels carefully and give each a try to see what works for you. Try these for "macaroni" and cheese too!

- Julienne zucchini, sauté briefly in garlic and butter or olive oil until soft... put Alfredo or homemade marinara on top with your favorite ingredients added.
- Kelp noodles are a great substitute and have a more pasta-like consistency after they sit and soak in a sauce overnight.
- Shirataki noodles are traditional Japanese noodles made from konjac flour, a water-soluble dietary fiber from the yam-like konjac plant.

Snacks

Think of an antipasto plate; cheese, meat, tree nuts, and green olives are perfect low-carb snacks. Here are some other crowd pleasers.

Low-carb veggies and high-fat dip

Be sure to NOT use low-fat dips or dressings! Full-fat sour cream and mayonnaise are the basis for veggie dip, then add spices like southwestern or Italian or dill. Add some tiny bits of pepperoni or ham perhaps. Think of the dip as the meal and the veggies as the vehicle.

Pepperoni poppers

Spread with a little cream cheese and fold over a pickled jalapeno. You could substitute pieces of green onion or crisp red pepper. The deli often has 2 or 3-inch diameter pepperoni and it's easier to work with, but the little ones are fun to eat. Do this with any deli meat!

Chip/cracker substitutes

You can dip any of these in just about anything you'd want… most dips are already low-carb. How about pub cheese, veggie dip, cream cheese dip, queso, artichoke dip, or French onion dip?

Be careful with salsa – ones from the store have sugar… sometimes quite a bit.

- Pepperoni as a chip. A thick cut works best.
  - ✓ Lay slices out on a cookie sheet and put in a 400-degree oven for just a few minutes until they get just a little crispy. Let them cool.
- Red pepper dippers. These are even better than the pepperoni for all around flavor. Cut red peppers in big enough pieces to be a scoop.
- Sliced raw zucchini and celery are also great chip substitutes.
- Fricos are fried cheese chips.
  - ✓ Google the term for recipes if you like. Basically, shred any type of cheese, put in small piles on a cookie sheet or frying pan, or make one big circle in a pan and then crack into chips when cooled. Cook until set and starting to lightly brown. You can even shape them before they cool if you act quickly.

Assignment for the week

1. Start your Personal Nutrition and Lifestyle Plan, and develop a tracking mechanism.
2. Grow your own your favorite foods list.
3. Track your intake, weigh at least 1x per week.
4. Learn more!
   - ✓ Consider starting to read one of the key resources noted in the Healthy Dimensions book. It can really help with motivation!
   - ✓ Explore message boards and forums on the Internet for tips, tricks, and recipes. (ActiveLowCarber.org forums are highly recommended, there are many others.)
   - ✓ When reading low-carb blogs and articles, always look for references to valid peer-reviewed professional research and not just opinions. The Internet is awash with nonsense and you're encouraged to look for evidence, not hype.

Growth Opportunities

This week we introduce a new kind of tool, Growth Opportunities. These include a variety of ways to enrich your experience, enhance motivation, and help you break through to a new level of power in your life. They include jumping-off points for self-exploration through journaling and various activities,

As with any tool in the HD program, these are completely optional.

You may wish to revisit these options after the intensity of the first few weeks has passed. Consider selecting one per week and add that goal to the lifestyle section of your PNLP. Check them off as you complete them.

Motivation builders
- ☐ Journal entry: Explore your goals. Not only your weight and size goals, but goals for the rest of your dimensions. How do you want to feel physically? What would you like to see change in your thinking and emotions?
- ☐ Journal entry: What will be the rewards of reaching a normal healthy weight? Think about the advantages both large and small; make a list as long as you can.

☐ Journal entry: Write about how your body feels as you go through the first week of low-carb eating.

Release the guilt about being overweight
☐ Journal entry: Write about how you've been told to lose weight in the past and how you feel about that. Write about the physiologic process you now know was happening in your body and forgive yourself.

Get organized for your new way of eating
☐ Exercise: Make a list of your favorite low-carb foods, plan the week's meals, go shopping, and restock your kitchen.
☐ Exercise: Make a list of your favorite foods and their carbohydrate content. Search the Internet for alternative low-carb recipes like cauliflower pizza crust. Try one!

Week 3 – Willpower   (HD Chapter 3)

Report out

How successful were you at following your Personal Nutrition and Lifestyle Plan (PNLP) last week?

What worked well?

What were the challenges and what did you do about them?

What is YOUR favorite new low-carb food?

Did you choose a Growth Opportunity? What did you learn?

Chapter content

How do you define willpower?

What would you say about your level of willpower?

How have your thoughts about yourself and the nature of willpower changed since reading this chapter?

Willpower and the depletion of mental energy

How does it feel inside your body when your mental energy is depleted?

Increased intensity of all emotions was the one consistent report when researchers asked people how it felt. What seems more intense when you're on empty?

Are there areas in life where you exercise a lot of willpower and other areas where you struggle? (For example, money, work, relationships, hobbies, tidiness, etc.)

1. Areas where willpower is strong:

2. Areas where willpower is weak:

Are there certain times or situations where your willpower around food is strong versus weak?

1. Times that are a struggle:

2. Situations that are a struggle:

What is it about these times or situations that may be depleting your mental energy for willpower?

Time or situation	What depletes my mental energy

Think about an event in the past where your mental energy was depleted and you overate. It might be a special event or even part of your routine, like eating cookies when you get home from work.

How might it have been different if you weren't depleted?

Consider the following key topics and choose one or more to spend some time with so you can learn how to become a Willpower Ninja! Don't worry, you don't have to do it all now. Revisit this section in the coming weeks and months to spend time with different tools.

Willpower tools

First and foremost are adequate nutrition, water, and sleep. Lack of these items will deplete your mental energy and ultimately your willpower around food.

Where or when do you find you may be pushing yourself and not getting enough?

Hydration:

Nutrition:

Sleep:

What are you willing to commit to regarding fatigue, hydration, and nutrition?

Explore and choose from the following Willpower Ninja tools and begin to develop lifestyle goals for your Personal Nutrition and Lifestyle Plan (PNLP) that will help you keep a full tank of mental energy and willpower!

Avoid temptation

Situations that create temptation:	Strategies: (include best sources of distraction)

Exercise willpower muscles

Research shows you can exercise your ability to have willpower and make it easier to prevent depletion.

Examples from research:
- Track your dietary intake.
- Use your non-dominant hand for 30 minutes a day.
- Speak without using um, uh, like, etc. or abbreviations like yeah, yup, nope.
- Stop using curse words.
- Spend 5 minutes a day doing something you don't really like to do but that is good for you or someone else.

Ways I might exercise willpower muscles:

Silence the inner nag

What are the sources of my inner nag?	What can I do to handle these sources?
How can I simplify and organize?	How can I create the time to handle my to-do list? (What are your time wasters?)

Make powerful goals

Review goals from Week 1, restate your primary goal here as powerful, long-term, and lofty. State it in the positive: I will...because...

Write or print this goal and post it in your personal environment, put it in your wallet...somewhere you're sure you see it regularly.

Who can you share these goals with to make them more public?

Who might be good cheerleaders?

A line in the sand: Boundaries

Write examples of certain specific boundaries that you think will be helpful to you in maintaining self-control with eating. As you design and institute your PNLP, think about diet/body-oriented boundaries as well as mental/emotional ones. When you discover one that is helpful, add it as a dietary or lifestyle goal in your tracking tool.

Suggested starters:

- I will always…

- I will never….

- I will only….

- If I….then I will

Make a plan: Clear and flexible

As you work on your PNLP and structure your meals, evaluate what you can do to make it a plan that is both clear AND flexible. This plan is for a lifetime, not just until you lose weight.

My clear and flexible plan for the upcoming week:

Share and compare

List 3 things you can do to create opportunities to network and share goals and efforts with others.

1.

2.

3.

Who could you ask to be an "observer" or buddy in the journey to healthy dimensions?

What will you do <u>this week</u> to create a buddy?

Self-awareness

What method will you use to track nutrition intake?

What method will you use to track your high-level Personal Nutrition and Lifestyle Plan goals?

I will weigh myself every_____

I will take my measurements every _____

Other things I will track:

Changing the food monolog

When there is a disconnect between your strongly held beliefs and standards for behavior and your actual actions, the primal emotional center sends out a chemical cascade to make you feel good (approach) or bad (avoid).

Close your eyes and imagine someone that you don't like very well. Then really vividly imagine poking them in the eye with a pen.

The uncomfortable feeling is your physiologic "avoid" response.

What does it feel like physically? Where?

When you notice that uncomfortable (avoid this) feeling, that means there is a primal emotional program running in your brain that will help drive actions. We want to use the known physiology of the brain to create clear standards (like "I really DO want to eat healthy") so that we have primal programs helping us instead of sabotaging us.

Setting clear standards: New beliefs I am adopting around food:

1.

2

3.

4.

Make a plan for changing the chatter in your mind about food

Develop messages to consciously send to your brain that support your new standards. Choose messages that guide your primal brain to feel perfectly fine, proud, and strong about missing out on a particular food. Be sure these messages relate to your goals! "I want this so I'm going to do that."

Messages I will say to my prefrontal cortex (PFC) when I'm facing a food challenge:

Praise I will say to my PFC about successfully turning down a food that's not on my plan:

Control stress chemicals

Whenever you feel physical tension in your body from stress or upset, breathe with a shorter inhalation and long, slow exhalation with pursed lips. This breathing reduces stress by activating the parasympathetic nervous system (PNS). Reducing stress increases mental energy for willpower. You can also practice this breathing technique at bedtime to quickly get deeply relaxed.

Write about the first time you use this technique to tone down the stress response here. What was the experience like?

Notice the negative bias of your brain

Each and every time you notice a negative thought, remind yourself that every human brain has a negative bias, and that it's not the real you. Inform your PFC with words (thought or spoken) that it is being overly cautious, negative, or fearful.

Three messages I will tell my PFC when I notice negative programs running in my head:

1.

2.

3.

This is not me, this is my creation

Recognize the real you, the one ultimately in control, is separate from the chatter in your head and the knee-jerk responses from the primal emotional brain center.

Complete this exercise:
1. Close your eyes and listen to the chatter in your head, really listen to the complexity and all the thoughts.
2. What emotion are you feeling in your body?
3. Then feel your body. Is it relaxed or tense?
4. Ask yourself, who is it that's listening and feeling?

This is the part of you that can guide the brain's programs and chatter. How would you describe this part of you that is the observer of the body and brain and that is really in charge?

As you start paying attention to the primal programs, identify instances where you can say
"This chatter in my head that is just the brain's negative bias. This is not me, this is a creation of my brain."

Chatter I notice that is simply a negative creation of my overcautious primal brain

Simulate success with food challenges

Participants in research studies on using simulation in the Alpha brainwave state were required to do this simulation daily, or at least several times a week. The research showed that the more often they did simulation, the better their results were.

Note 3 upcoming events during which it will be a challenge to stay on your nutrition plan. Pick at least one occurring in the next few days.

1.

2.

3.

Use the Healthy Dimensions Alpha Access Exercise recording named Success Simulation.

This recording is a guided relaxing experience lasting approximately 10 minutes. It will help you achieve the Alpha brainwave state and guide you in practicing simulation. Use one or more of your upcoming food challenges listed above as the focus.

While simulating:
✓ Use first person and simulate being inside yourself, not watching yourself
✓ Say actual words in your mind
✓ Include ALL senses while imagining the situation
✓ Include all emotions (feel the challenge of saying no as well as the pride)

After you do this a few times, you may become comfortable enough with the process to use one of the Alpha Access recordings without narration when you do simulation. Or you may prefer to practice simulation all on your own. Bedtime is a very natural time to practice simulation.

Describe your first experience with the simulation:

After the simulated event has passed, write about how things went and your level of willpower:

Is this a tool you wish to include in your PNLP? Why/why not?

TRACK simulating for success

Keep a record of simulation practice and results here.

Upcoming event	Dates the event was simulated	Outcome at event/comments

Assignment for the week

1. Complete your personal plan for the upcoming week. What will you include?
   - ✓ Dietary goals. Include any dietary changes you may make and recommit to tracking intake (it strengthens willpower muscles!)
   - ✓ Lifestyle goals. Make a goal to devote a certain number of minutes each day on your Healthy Dimensions process.
2. Spend the time you set aside with tools from this section that are a good fit for you. For example:
   - ✓ Be ready with messages to give your PFC about food
   - ✓ Post your powerful long-term lofty goal in places you will see it
   - ✓ Tell at least one person what your goals are
   - ✓ Consider selecting an "observer" or "buddy"
3. Do the Alpha State Success Simulation every day or nightly when you are ready for sleep.

Growth Opportunities

(always optional)

☐ Alpha State Exercise: What situations are the hardest for you to maintain control in and stick to your diet? Make a list of these situations. Choose one and do an Alpha Access simulation about going through that situation successfully. Repeat this situation or simulate others.

☐ Journal entry: Write yourself a pep talk about your PNLP and commitments to following it.

☐ Journal entry: Write about what YOU feel like when your mental energy is depleted (and your willpower is in jeopardy). What are the physical and emotional symptoms for you? This will help you identify these situations when they hit. What are some things in your life that you know deplete this well of energy?

☐ Exercise: Remove temptation, get all the unhealthy high-carb foods out of your home, car, and work area (or at least move them away from constant sight).

- ☐ Exercise: Make a list of all the things your inner nag has been reminding you of. Write a first step (only) for each and select a date when you will take that first step. Then, the next time you get nagged by brain voices, say "I don't have to worry about that now; I am worrying about that on ___."
- ☐ Exercise: Eliminate TV completely for a specified period of time (1 day if that's a lot to you) and substitute something that will quiet your inner nag or be fun and nurturing for you.
- ☐ Exercise: Make a commitment to getting at least 7 hours of sleep every night this week.
- ☐ Exercise: Pick an exercise to increase your willpower muscles. Suggestions: Keep excellent posture for a specified period of time, use your non-dominant hand, don't use words like "um" or "yeah," or do the Alpha Access exercise every day.
- ☐ Exercise: Awareness. If you aren't already, make a commitment to tracking your food intake consistently. If you eat something high in carbs, be sure to notice your body's response to this food.
- ☐ Journal entry: Review the weight loss goals you set. Create some intermediate goals or vital steps you will need to take. How can you make these goals long-term, lofty, or sacred and PUBLIC? Who can you share your goals with?
- ☐ Exercise: Pick a "diet buddy" and ask them to simply support your efforts; they don't have to do the program with you. Make a plan for regular check-ins about your progress and sticking with your commitments. Use the power of having an observer!
- ☐ Exercise: Make a list of boundaries you can establish that will make a clear line in the sand, so it becomes a "no brainer" and doesn't cost as much mental energy. For example, I will not eat ANY bread or pasta for one month. Or, I will have a green vegetable with dinner every night. Try putting some habit around your way of eating. For example, after dinner just make it your habit to not eat anything. Brush your teeth or chew some gum to remind you not to graze.
- ☐ Exercise: Put yourself in a challenging food situation at least once this week and have control and then journal about "How hard was it really?" Was it worth it?
- ☐ Exercise: For one meal, pay full attention and enjoy what you're eating. Savor every bite. Why do we do other things while we eat? Why do we eat fast? Change a message to "I deserve to enjoy this meal!" Consider doing this with every meal.

Week 4 – Food Sensitivities and Hunger-vs-Desire (HD Chapters 4 & 5)

Report out

How successful were you at following your Personal Nutrition and Lifestyle Plan (PNLP) last week?

What worked well?

What were the challenges and what did you do about them?

Did you choose a Growth Opportunity? What did you learn?

What willpower tools are you adopting?

Chapter content

What surprised you about these chapters?

What resonated with you the most?

What challenges you or even makes you feel uncomfortable?

Considering food sensitivities in your Personal Nutrition and Lifestyle Plan

Evaluate your health and family history for symptoms associated with chronic inflammation. Check the ones that are present.

☐ Joint and muscle pain
☐ Cognitive disorders (depression, anxiety, ADHD, schizophrenia, autism)
☐ Dizziness, muscle disorders (twitching, ALS, MS), seizures
☐ Memory problems (dementia, Alzheimer's)
☐ Peripheral nerve pain and problems
☐ Arteriosclerosis / hypertension
☐ Cancer
☐ Auto-immune disorders (rashes, acne, lupus, chronic fatigue, rheumatoid arthritis)

The most common symptoms of wheat sensitivity follow: Do you have any of these symptoms when you eat a big serving of chewy Italian bread or pasta?

☐ Symptoms of inflammation as described above
☐ Abdominal bloating/gas
☐ Abdominal pain and fullness
☐ Acid reflux/GERD or heartburn
☐ Diarrhea/constipation

More common food sensitivities include:

- Wheat/gluten
- Corn
- Soy
- Dairy
- Nightshades
- Artificial sweeteners

Do you think you may have a wheat/gluten sensitivity? Or other food sensitivity?

If you are concerned:

1. Learn more about food sensitivities and symptoms starting with the resources recommended in the Healthy Dimensions book.
2. Try eliminating highly allergenic foods and then reintroduce them with care, paying attention to effects on the body and mind. Do your research.
3. If you decide to consider testing for gluten sensitivity, research the options carefully before requesting a test.
    a. Genes: HLADQ2 and HLADQ8
    b. Antibody testing: Transglutaminase or endomysium are said to be more accurate than anti-gliadin. Endomysium detects only if you're still actively consuming wheat.

TRACK food sensitivity trails

Use this table (or another tracking format) to track any future trials of withholding and then reintroducing food types. If you discover one you are sensitive to, it will reduce inflammation in your body if you avoid it. You will feel better and lower your risk for chronic disease.

Food	Stop date	Response	Restart date	Response

Wheat and addictive exorphins

Be alert to cravings caused by eating wheat; its "morphine-like" exorphins affect receptors in everyone's brains. Exorphins are addictive, so they promote cravings.

When was the last time you ate wheat products?

If it has been two weeks or more, write about how your cravings have changed since the first day you went without it.

If you have not eliminated wheat, consider a trial.

You may think you can't live without it but each day cravings will get better, just like with any substance that is associated with these receptors. Use this table to track your response

Date I stopped eating wheat products____

Day	Level of craving 1-10	Comments
1		
2		
3		
4		
5		
6		

Day	Level of craving 1-10	Comments
7		
8		
9		
10		
11		
12		
13		
14		

When complete, come back and write about your experience of trying a wheat-free lifestyle:

Hunger vs. desire?

One of the ways a low carbohydrate diet works is that it encourages your body to burn your own fat. When it's doing that you won't be hungry as often.

If you eat when your body is trying to burn its own fuel, it will switch and burn the fuel you just gave it instead. Respecting true hunger and eating only until satisfied (not stuffed) is how you can lose weight without watching calories too closely.

Trust your body and work to adopt the belief "Food is just fuel." Say these words to your PFC every time you want to eat.

Keep it at the forefront of your mind. Create a sign for your refrigerator (or elsewhere) like this:

Am I hungry?
Food is just fuel
Go feed the need!

What does physical hunger feel like in your body?

How often do you "wanna eat" when you're not physically hungry?

Top 5 reasons "I wanna eat" when I'm not hungry:

1.

2.

3.

4.

5.

When you eat instead of managing the <u>situation</u> that makes you wanna eat, you are "stuffing it." Doing so can lead to allowing stressful and even damaging situations to continue. Are there situations in your life that you try to heal with food that really need to be addressed?

Things I have "stuffed" with food (or other escape mechanisms) instead of addressing them:

What are your thoughts and emotions around these things?

Feed the need: Awesome alternatives to food

Be ready with this list for the next time you want to eat but realize you're not really hungry.

What I can do to feed the needs instead:

<u>As rewards:</u>

1.

2.

3.

4.

5.

6.

7.

8.

9.

10.

For fatigue:

When bored:

Fun things to do:

1.

2.

3.

4.

5.

Things that would be nice to do for someone else:

1.

2.

3.

To handle something that's been nagging at me:

1.

2.

3.

Other awesome alternatives to eating when I'm not hungry:

TRACK I Wanna Eat log

Use this log or something similar for one week to track when you want to eat, your actual physical hunger level, and current mind/body state. Then add what you did and how that went.

I WANNA EAT log

Date	Time	Wanna eat (0-5)	Real hunger (-5 to +5)	Energy (-5 to +5)	Physical symptoms	Emotions/thoughts	Actions	Results

Write about what you learned with the "I Wanna Eat" log here:

End emotional eating: Changing your mind and choosing beliefs

Some things that make you "wanna eat" are emotional and harder to address than simple boredom or fatigue. There are certain steps you can take to gain control and end emotional eating.

Now that you are starting to understand how to use the PFC and ACC to control your primal emotional center and its knee-jerk responses, you can use this knowledge to reduce negative emotional states. The next step is to focus attention on the underlying beliefs that drive those primal emotional programs.

Basic steps to prevent end emotional eating:

1. **Pay attention**. Become conscious of the mental chatter, knee-jerk programs, and underlying beliefs that are driving the emotion.
2. **Either release it or reframe it**. Let it go, plan to think about it later, or tell your PFC a new story about it.
3. **Refocus on the here and now**. This step stops the chatter and knee-jerk emotional responses because <u>where you actively focus</u> drives the chemicals that create an emotional response.

The first dart of suffering is the actual pain that we all share in this life. The second dart of suffering we can control, which is our experience or story about what is actually happening.

Where is the second dart of suffering (how you choose to think about a situation) making your life more stressful?

Explore which beliefs could be changed to bring you more peace and power in your life. In the coming weeks and months, return to this table frequently when you notice programs and choose to eliminate the second dart by changing your story.

Current story about:	New story to tell my PFC
My self	
Food	
My weight	
My appearance	
What I deserve	
Health	
What I think I want	
What I think I need	
Other beliefs	

Programs and beliefs for future analysis

As you notice counterproductive or emotionally charged programs and chatter in your mind, explore how to attend to them: either by changing the situation or changing your mind.

- ✓ Handle what seems obvious.
- ✓ Start a list of those that need work – a "for future analysis" list. This action gives your brain permission to stop nagging you about it as long as you make an honest plan follow up later.
- ✓ Set a schedule to explore this list; your brain knows if you really are planning on addressing it. Even if you only devote 30 minutes a month, it sends the message.

Negative brain chatter and emotional responses	Underlying belief	Date to explore	Solution: Change the situation or change my mind

Assignment for the week

1. Update your PNLP goals while considering these things:
   - ✓ Are you going to change your nutrition plan for this week?
   - ✓ Are you willing to commit to the I Wanna Eat log for 1 week to see what's driving the desire when you're not really hungry?
2. Continue to grow your Awesome Alternatives to Eating list and when you are not hungry, feed the needs instead.
3. Focus drives feeling: practice focused attention in daily life (be here now).
   - ✓ Notice the chatter and programs running in your brain.
   - ✓ Shut them down when they are bugging you by paying full attention to what you're doing.
   - ✓ If you notice one returning regularly, you need to work on it. Add it to your list for future analysis to stop the constant reminders in your mind.
4. Make it easier for you to focus and be here now in your life: grow the focusing part of your brain by practicing focused attention in the Alpha state.
   - ✓ Use the Healthy Dimensions Alpha State Exercise recording Focused Attention or any commercially available meditation recording for developing mindfulness. You may also wish to simply use an un-narrated recording or no recording at all.
   - ✓ If you want results, doing it daily is best.
   - ✓ Bedtime is a great time to do this exercise; the programs and thoughts can get really loud when you want to go to sleep.
   - ✓ You may want to combine willpower simulation with focusing your attention. Just make the extra step of noticing when your mind wanders and really focus on the process of simulation.

Growth Opportunities

(always optional)

☐ Exercise: Draw a picture of the primal/emotional part of yourself that wants to be loved and nurtured and protected and listened to. Include its surroundings, what it's saying to you and about you. Write a note to this part of you, acknowledging it and stating what you will start doing to provide comfort and joy.

- ☐ Journal entry: How did you feel about the above experience?
- ☐ Journal entry: Write about your relationship with hunger. What new messages can you give yourself about the nature and meaning of hunger?
- ☐ Exercise: When did food and/or your weight become an issue in your life? Was it just slowly over many years, or was your weight gain relatively quick? Create a graph of your weight changes throughout your life, labeling it with primary life issues or milestones. Are there life events or patterns of emotions that you think are more associated with your weight?
- ☐ Journal entry: Write about any correlations you saw in the preceding exercise and how you can use this knowledge to affect your success with achieving healthy dimensions now.
- ☐ Journal entry: Review your hunger log. How did you do? Count how many times you did change your mind and decide to not eat. Did you stop when you were satisfied? Write some praise to yourself and about how you might handle an individual situation differently in the future.
- ☐ Journal entry: Finish the statement "I worry that if I were thin I would…" with as many endings as you can think of. Then evaluate them from your higher intellectual self and evaluate how rational or irrational these are. Then finish the statement "If I were thin people might…" Re-examine your previous list about the rewards of losing weight and see if there is a dark side that might be driving a fear of losing weight. Is there something about being overweight that is beneficial (less romantic attention, lower expectations in work/life)? Does being overweight make us somehow different (which can be "special")?
- ☐ Journal entry: Contemplate hunger and the meanings that you have attached to that physiologic feeling.
- ☐ Exercise: New rules, such as just because you cook dinner doesn't mean you have to eat it – or you don't have to eat when everyone else does – or every meal doesn't have to be a production (looking for a special occasion or "I deserve this because").
- ☐ Journal entry: What are some reasons that you think you need to have a special food treat? For example, just finished five 10-hour days of work, finished a big project… or the sun came up today. Be prepared by making a list of alternative rewards and ways to view food as just fuel.
- ☐ Exercise: Try making dinner a non-production, something simple and quick but satisfying. Does dinner always have to be an event? Is there an opportunity to de-emphasize eating somewhere in your life? What time would you have available to do something else you love if you weren't making big fancy meals?
- ☐ Exercise: Identifying hunger – draw a picture of where you feel things when you are hungry. Next time you're really hungry, compare and improve on the image. Think about what these

feelings are and change your thinking that this is the only message you should be responding to with food.

☐ Exercise: Pick a day you'll be home or where food will be available but not ubiquitous, let yourself get truly hungry, and then eat something quite small, like ¼ of a meal and wait to see how long it takes for hunger to return. What does it feel like to just remove the hunger without getting "stuffed" by a big meal? Identify what it feels like to just be satisfied and not full.

☐ Journal entry: Note your physiological responses and also what you're saying to yourself about the above experience in your journal.

☐ Exercise: For one day, carry a piece of paper and put a mark for every negative thought about your body, weight, eating, other people, or situations. How many times? Imagine the mental freedom and confidence you would have without all this internal criticism? It is natural for the brain to go negative. Start working on some alternate beliefs to replace the negatives when they show up.

☐ Journal entry: The first dart of suffering is out of your control, but the second dart of feelings and emotions is under your control. Write about something, a situation or a memory that makes you suffer, and how you can change your story about it.

Week 5 – Stress and Choosing Beliefs (HD Chapter 6)

Report out

What challenges did you have with your PNLP this week?

What successes did you have?

What did you discover from noticing the programs running in your brain?

How did focusing on what you're doing here and now help with the chatter in your head?

What did you learn from the "I Wanna Eat" log?

Chapter content

What surprised you about this chapter?

What resonated with you the most?

How stressed out do you feel?

Do you think stress is affecting your health? How?

What do you think about the concepts and tools discussed to reduce stress?

Identifying the stress response

Reducing stress helps with emotional eating and is healthier in general. Explore stress in your life.

Identify your stress response: write about what that feels like physically:

How to change the physiology:
The chemical cascade that causes the physical stress response can be inhibited by stimulating the parasympathetic nervous system (PNS) simply by breathing a certain way. Relatively short or normal inhale and slow exhale through pursed lips.

Notice your current state of tension. Give it a number 1-10 _____

Now close your eyes and use this breathing technique for 2 or 3 breaths

Can you feel the difference?

How often do you feel a full blown the stress response?

TRACK the stress response

Start to use this log daily to write about the effects on your body

Event	Physical effects & response to stimulating PNS (physical & emotional)

Identifying stressors

What are the major stressors in your life?

1.

2.

3.

4.

5.

Things that have me do-do-doing all the time:

1.

2.

3.

4.

5.

What does do-do-doing all the time give you?
(For example, pride, money, appreciation, compliments)

Situations where I will start saying no:

Things I choose to get organized:

What will it take for you to get organized in these areas?

Ways I can simplify my life to remove stressors:

What would I give up if I simplified in these ways?

Should-ing on yourself and powerful choices

Notice every time you use the words "I should" and explore how to:
1. Dump it if you don't really want to do it or believe it...life is too short to do things you really don't want to do. And doing them will make you want to eat as a reward!
2. If it is something you HAVE to do, make it into a true and powerful choice instead.
3. Use the word choice or choose when referring to this situation in your mind and out loud to other people. (For example, I choose to do this because if I didn't....)

Things I should on myself about	My powerful choice

More things I should on myself about	My powerful choice

Changing your mind about stressors

1. **Notice it's happening** (wow, I'm really stuck ruminating about this thing)
2. **Depersonalize** (it's not me, it's the negative bias of the human primal brain)
3. **Activate the PNS** (breathe with a slow exhale through pursed lips)
4. **Release it** (this is not worth losing my health over, I'm letting it go for now)
5. **Reframe it** (this is not as bad as my brain and its negative bias thinks)
6. **Refocus** (on what you're doing right now)

Use this space to begin documenting the things you'd like to change your mind about. Write out at least three things now that bug you and how you'll change your mind. As you pay attention to the programs running in your brain, return to this list and add them. Make a plan for how you will respond when you notice them.

Things I notice bugging me and negative chatter in my mind	Words I will say to my PFC to release and reframe

More things I notice bugging me and negative chatter in my mind	Words I will say to my PFC to release and reframe

Work through tough stressors – Dig into beliefs

Sometimes it's clear and easy to know what you need to do to stop the negative chatter and programs running in your mind about a particular stressor (for example, just say no).

For the more difficult situations, a process is provided here to stop stress-producing chatter and programs. This logical process helps you:

- ✓ identify the beliefs to examine
- ✓ make powerful choices
- ✓ develop new messaging for your PFC

When you make conscious choices about your beliefs, you drive your experience instead of being blown about by the changing winds of life.

Work through this process each time you identify a tough stressor. It may take only a few minutes or it may require more time. You might want to identify areas where you want the support of a friend or counselor to make tough, lasting changes in what you choose to believe.

Identify the beliefs underlying the stressor:
Stressor:
Beliefs I hold that actually make this stressful: (such as it shouldn't be this way, it isn't fair, I want something else more etc.)

List the potential outcomes from holding these beliefs: (positive and negative)

Because I believe this I get to...

Because I believe this I am pushed to...

List the potential outcomes from discarding these beliefs: (positive and negative)

If I stop believing this I don't have to....

If I stop believing this I will be pushed to...

Make your choices and take control
Counterproductive beliefs I am discarding and why:
Empowering beliefs I am choosing about this from now on are:
Should I avoid it? Fix it? Or change my mind?
Actions I am choosing:
Words I can say to my PFC about this situation (use your new empowering beliefs):

TRACK progress on stress

In the coming weeks you will identify beliefs or situations that are causing a stress response in your body. Return to this list in the weeks and months to come. Work on one stressor at a time.

Things that produce a stress response in my body	What I can do about it

Love yourself

Say the words <u>out loud</u> "I love myself" 3 times (really, do it).

Describe what you felt in your body when you said that?

Describe your emotions when you said it?

What do you say to yourself when you look in the mirror?

Unkind things I say about myself that I wouldn't say to a friend, or even a stranger:

Make a commitment to treat yourself with the same respect you pay to people who you love. Correct yourself every time you do so!

5 ways that I can treat myself with love and respect and kindness:

1.

2.

3.

4.

5.

TRACK how often you are good to yourself

Date	Loving thought, word, or deed and how that felt

Assignment for the week

1. Update your PNLP with nutrition and lifestyle changes you've chosen.
2. Practice once with the Alpha State Exercise recording Powerful Life.
   - ✓ Continue to use Powerful Life or use one of the other Alpha state tools you've learned.
3. When you are deprogramming stress and you tell your PFC "I will think about that later," return here and continue adding to your lists for awareness and accountability.
   - ✓ Set a date and time to explore it....doing so helps stop the nagging reminders.
4. For one week, treat yourself like you would a friend visiting your home: love yourself in thought, word, and deed.

Growth Opportunities

(always optional)

- ☐ Exercise: For one day, make a commitment to noticing every time you use the word *should* and change it to *will*, *can*, or *choose to* (or *choose not to*). Do this in your head as well as out loud.
- ☐ Journal entry: List 5 major "shoulds" that you lay on yourself. Examine whether you will drop them or turn them into choices.
- ☐ Journal entry: If you are over-busy and over-committed, make a list of all the things you could potentially say no to that you usually say yes to. Write out HOW you would say no in these situations and how it would feel to release that responsibility.
- ☐ Exercise: Once this week, say NO to something that you could do but don't really WANT to do. See how that feels. Were the consequences less severe than you imagined? How did you feel afterwards? Ready to pick something else to get off your plate?
- ☐ Exercise: Make a list of things you want to do or get handled, the things driving your inner nag. Set a date and time to address each of these things, even if it's weeks into the future, and post the list where you can see it and be reminded of your commitment.
- ☐ Journal entry: Write about how you might simplify your life and how that might look and feel. Consider the pros and cons for you and others in your world.
- ☐ Exercise: Is your environment chaotic? Organize something, then take time to appreciate how great it feels to have that handled.

- ☐ Journal entry: Your story. Distilled down, your life story is just a story; how do you choose to interpret all that has gone before? Write down how you usually tell your story (to yourself or others). Then, write a new version of the story in which you're lovable, did the best you could and so did everybody else, given their baggage.
- ☐ Exercise: See the previous journal entry. Instead, tell the old story and the new story to someone.
- ☐ Journal entry: Childhood programs. We are most impressionable and create foundational brain programs in childhood. Examine the programs around body image, food, and weight that may have started in childhood. Use the Deprogramming stress worksheet to determine the best way to change the program. What new message will you give to your PFC? Add this to your Change My Mind list.
- ☐ Journal entry: What messages have you been giving yourself about your body? Take a look at those who were closest to you growing up (family/friends/teachers). What attitudes did they have about their own bodies? Have you taken on some of their messaging? How can you change these messages and forgive them by owning your own body attitudes? Add them to your Change My Mind list.
- ☐ Journal entry: Look in the mirror at your body (yes, naked). What messages do you hear yourself saying? Are these messages based on something someone else said or did? Are you comparing yourself to some unreasonable ideal? Write down these messages and how you can revise them. Add these to your Change My Mind list.
- ☐ Journal entry: Feel your personal power. Think of a time when you achieved a really hard goal, a real physical or emotional challenge. What did you do to get through this experience? How did you feel when you succeeded – did you feel powerful? Take yourself there and re-experience it – acknowledge yourself for being awesome… write down the sensations you feel in your body.
- ☐ Exercise: See the previous journal entry. Complete this process in Alpha state practice.

Week 6 – Inflammation and Happiness (HD Chapters 7 & 8)

Report out

What challenges did you have with your PNLP?

What successes did you have?

What tools are you using to change your relationship with food, reduce stress, change your mind and make powerful choices?

When looking back to when you started this process, what are you pleased about so far?

Chapter content

What resonated with you in these chapters?

What surprised you?

What challenged you?

Do I have chronic inflammation?

A C-Reactive protein blood test will help point to chronic inflammation somewhere in the body, but it is not very specific. Consider the following risk factors.

Chronic inflammation is thought to be a root cause of many degenerative diseases such as:
- Heart disease
- Cancer
- Diabetes
- Autoimmune disorders (Rheumatoid arthritis, eczema, psoriasis)
- Cirrhosis and fatty liver disease
- Depression
- Cognitive decline (memory problems, dementia and Alzheimer's)

Do you have any of these disorders now?

Apple-shaped people are more likely to have chronic inflammation than pear-shaped people because visceral fat (in the abdomen) generates inflammatory chemicals.

> What is your waist measurement? _____
> What is your hip measurement? _____
> Divide the waist measurement by the hip measurement _____

A waist/hip ratio above .9 for men and .85 for women is considered abdominal obesity and is associated with increased inflammation.

Blood sugar spikes promote inflammation; high fructose corn syrup (HFCS) is particularly pro inflammatory. Any human will have a blood sugar spike if they eat a big enough carb load.

Before you changed your way of eating, do you think you were promoting inflammation from frequent carb loads?

When insulin rises, leptin rises, which promotes inflammation in the body that often manifests as pain in joints.

Did you have painful joints? Where?

Have they improved from lowering your carb intake and circulating insulin?

Leptin also signals the brain to create strong feelings of hunger. Decreased hunger suggests decreased leptin and therefore inflammation.

How have your cravings and hunger changed?

Did you or do you eat a lot of vegetable oils (high omega-6) or margarine and partially hydrogenated vegetable shortening (trans fats)?

Do you think you are at risk for chronic inflammation?

Why or why not?

Reversing inflammation

Ways to reverse chronic inflammation

1. De-stress our lives
2. Low-carbohydrate food and NO HFCS!
3. Identify food sensitivities
4. Fats to enjoy
    -   Saturated – lard, butter, coconut oil
    -   Monounsaturated – olive, avocado, palm, almond oils
5. Fats to avoid
    -   Margarine or shortening with trans fats
    -   Oils with high % omega 6 fatty acids (such as safflower, sunflower, corn, soybean)
6. Eat omega 3-rich seafood, meats, and eggs
7. Add turmeric and fresh garlic to foods

Changes I could consider to decrease my risk of chronic inflammation:

Alcohol

How has your alcohol consumption changed since you started this program?

What have you noticed about that?

Is it harder to stay on your nutrition plan when you drink alcohol?

Are you more likely to "give up for today" and get out of control with eating?

If/when you have reintroduced alcohol to your PNLP, pay close attention and track your body's response. Some people can enjoy the occasional cocktail and continue to lose weight, some cannot.

TRACK response to alcohol

Date	Type & Amount	Response: Weight x 3 days, changes in hunger or cravings?

Happiness

On a scale of 1-10 with 10 being constantly elated and zero being catatonically depressed, where does your baseline happiness reside?

What have you always thought would make you happier?

Evidence suggests we can all increase happiness by choosing to do more of these things, do you believe this is possible?

Why or why not?

Gratitude

How often do you take the time to feel gratitude?

When was the last time you expressed gratitude to someone else?

Try this 5-minute gratitude exercise:

3 things I'm grateful for that happened today:
1.

2.

3.

3 things I'm grateful for that happened this month:
1.

2.

3.

3 things I'm grateful for that happened in the last few years:
1.

2.

3.

3 things I'm grateful for in my life as a whole:
1.

2.

3.

Optimism

People are not born optimists or pessimists. Optimists choose to view experiences differently than pessimists. Research suggests you can become optimistic by seeing unfortunate situations as:

- ✓ **Isolated** (this doesn't REALLY happen all the time)
- ✓ **External** (this really is about someone else and their problems, it's not about me)

When misfortune great or small rears its ugly head, always consider both points of view.

- ✓ Start with one fairly minor thing that happened in the last 48 hours (for example, your computer crashed) and write the optimistic perspective.
- ✓ Say these words in your mind so your PFC hears you and shuts off the negative chemical cascade in your body.
- ✓ Come back and work more on finding the optimistic view.

Misfortune	Pessimist: Global and internal view	Optimist: Isolated and external view

Create flow experiences

What are the top 3 activities that give you the "flow" experience? (Generally noted by intense concentration, positive challenge, and rapid passage of time)

1.

2.

3.

You deserve to do what you love. It is a perfect way to "feed the need" when you're not sure what the need is but it makes you wanna eat.

How can you reorder your life to allow time for yourself to experience flow?

What are the biggest time wasters in your life?

Some common ones:
- ☐ Surfing the internet
- ☐ Social networking
- ☐ TV / video entertainment or games
- ☐ Spending time with people who you don't really enjoy
- ☐ Shopping for things you don't really NEED

How much time can you create each day by reducing or eliminating your time wasters?

Make a commitment!
I will do _____ less
I commit to giving myself _____ hours each week to create flow in my life by _____

Schedule this time on your calendar and put it on your PNLP.

Assignment for the week

1. Make changes to your Personal Nutrition and Lifestyle Plan for the upcoming week.
2. Choose one happiness exercise from the Get Happy! Growth Opportunities list for this week.
3. Practice an Alpha State Exercise with the Gratitude recording.
4. Continue to practice the Alpha State exercises that work best for you, with or without recordings. (Simulation for success, Focused Attention training, living a Powerful Life, and Gratitude)

Growth Opportunities

Get happy!

Gratitude
- ☐ Once a week, spend 10 minutes writing about what you're grateful for from the previous week.
- ☐ Once a week, spend your Alpha Access time focusing on gratitude.
- ☐ Write a letter to someone to express gratitude.
- ☐ Pay a visit to someone to express gratitude.

Being helpful
- ☐ Pick a day for random acts of kindness. On that day, go out of your way to help a stranger at least 3 times.
- ☐ Pick a task that a friend, coworker, or family member usually does and offer to do it.
- ☐ Make and keep a commitment to volunteer somewhere.

Optimism
- ☐ Pay attention for pessimistic thoughts and attitudes.
- ☐ Change your perspective from global to isolated and from a personal cause to an external cause. Keep track of your progress!
- ☐ If one of them is hard to change, add it to your list of things you want to change your mind about and spend some time on alternate messages when time allows.

Stop overthinking

☐ For one day, commit to "be here now" as much as possible. You will be surprised at how little time you spend here now.

☐ Practice simple mindfulness during Alpha state exercise on a daily basis to strengthen the ability to refocus on the task at hand.

Avoid social comparisons

☐ Spend one day really attending to how often you compare yourself and your life to others and write them down.

☐ Make a list of all the ways you compare yourself to others. Ask yourself, on a scale of 1 to 10, how important will these things be when you look back at your life on your dying day. Then, make a list of the things that will matter on that day.

☐ When you find yourself making a social comparison, immediately refocus on something you're happy you've made a priority in your life.

Forgiveness

☐ Write a letter. Work through all the wrongs that were done to you, then try to empathize with the offender (include any role you may have had) and state your forgiveness. (You can deliver it, tuck it away to re-read, or burn it in a ritual; as the smoke rises, let your anger float away with it.)

☐ Use Alpha Access time to imagine opening your heart to the buried good in that person.

☐ If you want to heal the relationship, have a conversation with the person after writing down the main points that you want to make.

☐ For profoundly painful situations, consider reading one of the many good books on forgiveness or working with a counselor.

Savor the good

☐ For one day, make a commitment to look for beauty everywhere. When your mind is reeling about something, STOP and look around you. A flower, a lovely child, the sky, the heavy gray of clouds. Savor the beauty around you for one day. Then maybe do it again.

☐ For one day, when someone says or does something nice, SAVOR it. Don't deflect it. Stop, wait a few seconds to let it sink in, and then say thank you. In fact, remember it later and savor it again. Make it emotional to get those neurons to fire and wire together and form positive implicit memories and brain chemicals.

- ☐ Start a compliment journal and write them down every time you get one.

Flow activities

- ☐ Continue your list of things that put you in a flow state. Reach into your past and think about things you used to do but don't anymore.
- ☐ Make a commitment to include flow activities in place of time wasters in your life.

Grow a social network

- ☐ List 3 people you'd like to have a stronger relationship with, and list 3 things you could do to enhance each relationship. Or, list 3 ways you could meet new people.
- ☐ Each week, plan at least one activity to get you around people who share something in common with you. Be open to the potential for genuine friendships to develop.
- ☐ Determine a realistic schedule for seeing or speaking with existing friends to keep them close in your heart and reach out to them in that timeframe if they haven't already reached out to you

Set goals

- ☐ Make a list of all goals you had when you were younger but never pursued. Cross out any that don't interest you anymore. Brainstorm about other small and large things you'd like to do or achieve. Pick one small goal and one big one. Write a high-level plan for achieving the goals. Then write what you're going to do tomorrow to start.
- ☐ What can you get excited about? If you had unlimited time, what would you do with it (besides travel to exotic places...eventually you'd get tired of that). What would be the most fun or rewarding things? List 5 in order of importance. Pick one and list 3 "first steps" you could do in the next week toward this thing.

Physical options

- ☐ Move your body in whatever way sounds like FUN.
- ☐ Make walking or other exercise a meditation on love and appreciation for your body. "My legs are perfect and move me forward, my arms are strong." Make a big mental deal when you're done about how good you feel, change the message in your head to "I feel good" rather than "I've met my promise but I didn't want to." Describe how you feel after some exercise.

- [ ] Consider a 5-minute walk whenever you have some abstract need that you can't identify (it may show up as "I wanna eat"). If the walk seems to satisfy it you, then you may have discovered your "move me" voice!
- [ ] Smile – every single time you think of it, all day long, even when you're alone.
- [ ] Laugh – watch funny movies, read funny things on the web, hang out with funny people. Make a plan to schedule things that will make you laugh if you don't have some good belly laughs every day.
- [ ] Hug – if this is not a regular part of your life then start creating it. You can even hug animals.

Week 7 – Maintaining a Healthy Relationship with Food (HD Chapter 9)

Report out

What successes and challenges did you have with your Personal Nutrition and Lifestyle plan this week?

What has been the most helpful for you in this Healthy Dimensions program?

What do you think about using the tools you've learned about in this program to change your relationship with food?

What tools do you now have on your PNLP?

What tools are you thinking of revisiting later?

Chapter content

What was helpful about this chapter?

What surprised you?

What challenged you?

Planning for favorite foods

You may choose to completely eliminate some foods, but if you want to have some of them on occasion you need to plan for it. Use this list to be aware of the nutritional profile of your favorite foods. See what the NET carbs in a full serving are. Also calculate how much of that food would be just 5 grams of NET carbs.

If you set the belief that you can be happy with a 5-gram serving, you can add this back into your way of eating without fear of stimulating insulin and ultimately cravings.

Food	NET carb grams in regular serving	Size of 5 gram NET carb serving
1		
2		
3		
4		
5		
6		
7		
8		
9		
10		
11		
12		
13		
14		
15		
16		
17		
18		
19		
20		

TAME a binge

What does "a binge" mean to you?

What does "a binge" feel like physically?

What does "a binge" feel like emotionally?

Write about the last time you felt out of control with food and why you think it happened:

When things start to feel out of control, remember:

- **T is for Take a breath**. The moment you start to feel out of control, stop and take a breath. Literally take a few slow breaths and try to get your parasympathetic nervous system (PNS) activated and your body relaxed (quick inhale and slow exhale through pursed lips).

- **A is for Awareness**. Bring your awareness to the present moment and what is going on for you... body, mind, and emotions. How does your body feel? What have you actually eaten? As soon as possible, write all your intake down honestly and then figure out the nutritional profile as soon as practical. This is accountability in action. It will make you feel stronger for keeping your commitment to tracking.

- **M is for Move**. Move away from the source of food.

- **E is for Enjoy and evaluate**. Find something to do that you really enjoy or at least something that is distracting. See if you can determine the trigger for the out-of-control eating.

Change your mind about what just happened
- ✓ Own the choice
- ✓ Stop beating yourself up
- ✓ Focus on your strengths
- ✓ This is a physiologic response to excess insulin

Return to fat metabolism

- Fast until actual hunger returns. Drink plenty of water; your body wants to retain it.
- Recommit to VERY low carb for a few days. Emphasize fat over protein to keep insulin low. No alcohol until successfully in fat metabolism.
- If your nutrition plan includes watching total calories, don't worry about them for a couple of days. Focus on real hunger and feeding the real needs.
- Water loss occurs 2-3 days after a carb load. This may increase potassium and sodium needs, so be alert for symptoms (see Week 2).
- Track all intake. Awareness is an important willpower tool and creates accountability in your brain.
- Weigh daily until you are losing again to learn your body's responses.

Use the power of an observer

Explore these alone or with a "buddy" (even by email).
1. What I ate (# cal, carb)

2. Reason for making that choice

3. Where did it go off the rails metabolically and kick in the cravings?

4. What I did for distraction to fight the cravings and stop the binge

5. How I feel

6. What I learned

7. What I will do next time...

Get a buddy!

Who could you ask to be your buddy, the person you report to about your progress and challenges in the coming weeks as you drive toward your goals?

What will you do to use this relationship to strengthen your commitment to your plan? (Scheduled calls? Emails?)

Planning for the rest of the journey

Set realistic goals

Looking like a super model is not required for joy and love in this life. Being healthy enough to feel good and do all the things you want to do is required. Recent research has suggested being at the low end of the "overweight" BMI category may even be healthier than being at the low end of "normal." Listen to your body and find the balance.

1. Your body's healthiest weight may not be what you think it is.
2. Don't expect to lose more than 1-2 pounds per week, even if you adhere to your plan.
   - Menstrual cycles always affect weight, don't freak out.
   - If you eat a carb load, it will likely take 3 days to return to the previous weight even if you adhere to your plan.
3. Don't expect to be perfect. When you fall off the wagon, just keep getting back on. Do the TAME process. Get support, get a buddy.

Fine-tune your nutrition plan

1. Add additional grams of carb if desired
   - Increase by ~5 grams per day for a full week. Some people are most comfortable staying around 20 grams NET carb.
   - Weigh yourself at least weekly. If you have lost weight, consider another increase of 5 grams or just stay where you are.
   - Ask yourself, am I starting to have cravings and hunger again? If so, evaluate and reduce carbs until the cravings recede.
2. Split carbohydrate servings over the day to reduce blood sugar and insulin spikes.
3. When you reach your comfortable weight loss rate, hover around that level of carbohydrates.
   - As you approach your goal, things may change.
   - Your perfect level is not always the same. Your body will tell you. Return to tracking if you stray far from goal.
4. Try to reintroduce foods one at a time to better see how your body reacts to them.
   - Be aware of any signs of inflammation or intolerance (joints, belly, head, skin).

- Ask "Which foods make me feel vital?" and "Which make me feel sluggish or uncomfortable in other ways?"
5. Eat to satisfy hunger, food is fuel. If you just wanna eat, ask yourself:
   - How am I adding pleasure other than food to my life?
   - How am I stretching and growing?
   - How do I need to change my mind and enjoy this moment without a food treat?
6. If you are not losing, consider evaluating your caloric intake.
   - Sometimes, setting a calorie target makes you pay closer attention to whether you are really hungry.
   - Calories do count for some people. The good news is you won't feel starving at that lower calorie level because you are reducing insulin and leptin!
   - You need to pay attention to feeding the real needs.

Continue to develop your PNLP

1. Continue with those practices that support a calm mind, lack of stress, and joy in life. Revisit this workbook regularly to try new tools such as:
   - Growth Opportunities: Journaling/exercises
   - Alpha state exercises for simulation and focused attention
   - Changing your mind and reducing stress to end emotional eating
   - Developing a higher happiness baseline

2. Establish and maintain a lifestyle support network
   - If you don't already have a buddy to share your plans and "report in" with, it's time to do that now.
   - Network online with other Healthy Dimensions program participants.
   - Invite friends to do the program with you, be their buddy as they walk through the first 6 weeks.

3. Come back to this workbook and continue to grow all of your dimensions. Carry on with the journey to realizing your dream of being a healthy weight and living a life you love!

Creating an ongoing support group

What would you like to get from a support group?

If you are doing this program with a group (or have decided to create one), take some time to consider the following for the coming weeks and months:

Structure for ongoing support meetings

What is our mission statement?

Schedule
- How often will we meet?

- How long are the meetings?

- What days/times are best?

What is the best way to give all a chance to attend at least some?

- What are good locations?

Structure
- Is there a basic structure we want to use with certain things always included?

- What are some ideas for other things/topics to include?

Planning
- How will we decide who is leading each meeting?

- Who decides what the meeting will include?

- How will we be sure everyone gets a chance to contribute during the meeting?

- What method will we use for logistical planning?

- Do we want to host open meetings for other grads?

First meeting
- Date/time
- Location
- Leader
- Structure

How will we network online to give/receive support?

Make a list of potential excursions

Ideas for ongoing support meetings

Healthy Dimensions strongly recommends allowing time for reporting out on personal plans, successes, and challenges. Doing so is critical for accountability, which is one of the most important purposes of the group.

Consider creating a time to:
- Review various exercises people may have done from those provided in the Healthy Dimensions materials (revisit exercises, do a new growth opportunity each week, etc.)
- Develop new exercises that are meaningful to the group and then discuss outcomes on forums or at a subsequent meeting.
- Feature "latest research" and explore new concepts and studies critically.

Consider putting general topics on cards in a fishbowl and selecting one or more to discuss.

You can do it!

Thank you for giving yourself the gift of this powerful process for life transformation.

This is only the beginning. You will spend the coming months discovering exactly what nutrition and lifestyle changes will make weight loss perfectly natural for you.

You will start making powerful choices and driving your experience of life, instead of letting life drive your experience.

You are redesigning your approach to living (not just eating) and you will be amazed at how wonderful it can be.

We believe in you, you can do it!

Please share your feedback and let us know about your progress.
- Via the website: Healthy-Dimensions.com
- Via email: Administrator@Healthy-Dimensions.com
- Via Facebook: www.facebook.com/healthydimensionsweightloss

Stay in touch!

The Healthy Dimensions team

www.ingramcontent.com/pod-product-compliance
Lightning Source LLC
Chambersburg PA
CBHW081107290526
45795CB00006B/2029